Diabetic Diet Easy Cookbook

Don't Miss These Quick and Easy Recipes to Make Incredible Keto Diet Appetizers

Roseann Smith

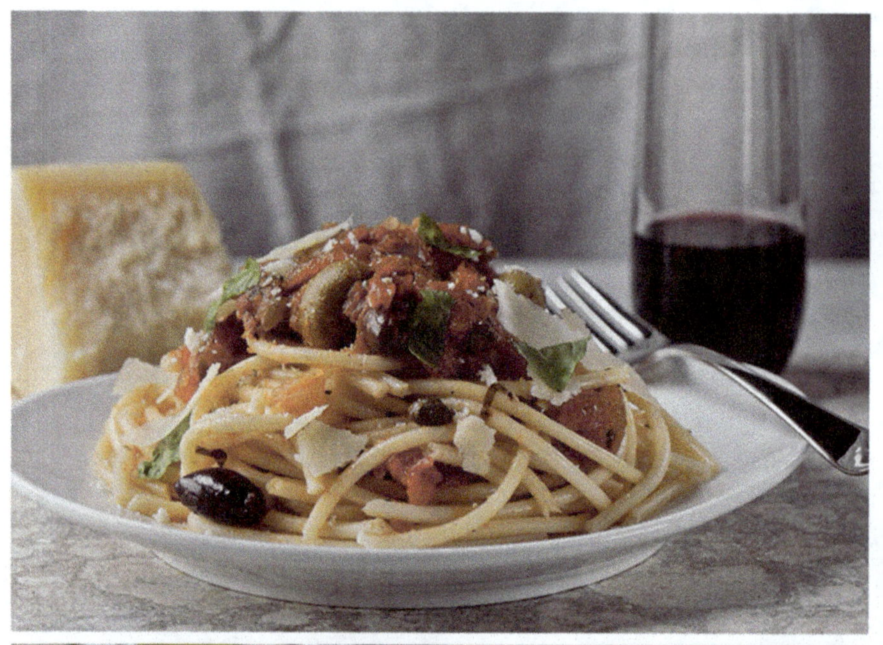

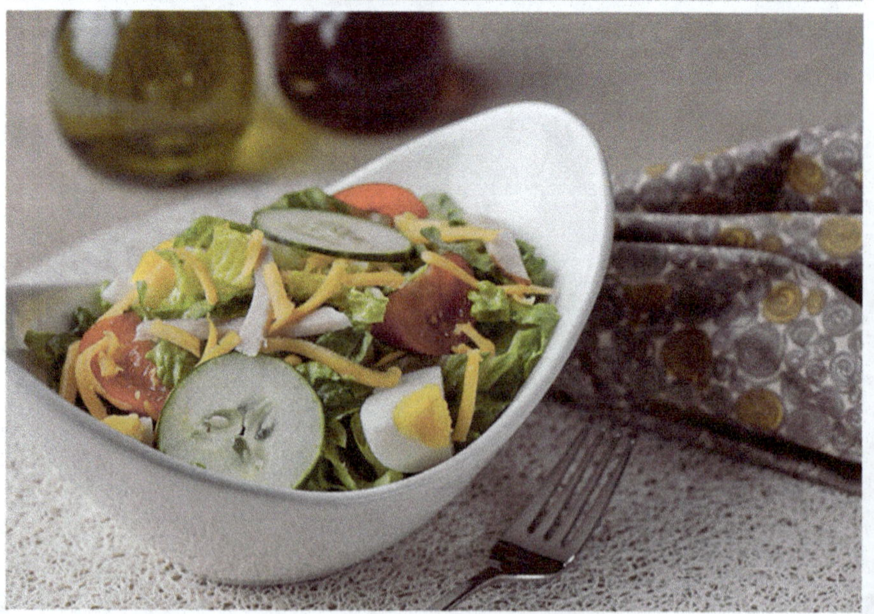

Disclaimer Notice:

Please note the information contained within this document is for educational and entertainment purposes only. All effort has been executed to present accurate, up to date, and reliable, complete information. No warranties of any kind are declared or implied. Readers acknowledge that the author is not engaging in the rendering of legal, financial, medical or professional advice. The content within this book has been derived from various sources. Please consult a licensed professional before attempting any techniques outlined in this book.

By reading this document, the reader agrees that under no circumstances is the author responsible for any losses, direct or indirect, which are incurred as a result of the use of information contained within this document, including, but not limited to, — errors, omissions, or inaccuracies.

Table of Contents

Tomato Risotto

Servings: 4

Cooking Time: 30 Minutes

Ingredients:

- 1 cup shallots, chopped
- cups cauliflower rice
- tablespoons olive oil
- cups veggie stock
- 1 cup tomatoes, crushed
- ¼ cup cilantro, chopped
- ½ teaspoon chili powder
- 1 teaspoon cumin, ground
- 1 teaspoon coriander, ground

Directions:

1. Heat up a pan with the oil over medium heat, add the shallots and sauté for 5 minutes.
2. Add the cauliflower rice, tomatoes and the other ingredients, toss, cook over medium

heat for 25 minutes more, divide between plates and serve.

Nutrition Info: Calories 200 Fat 4 Fiber 3 Carbs 6 Protein 8

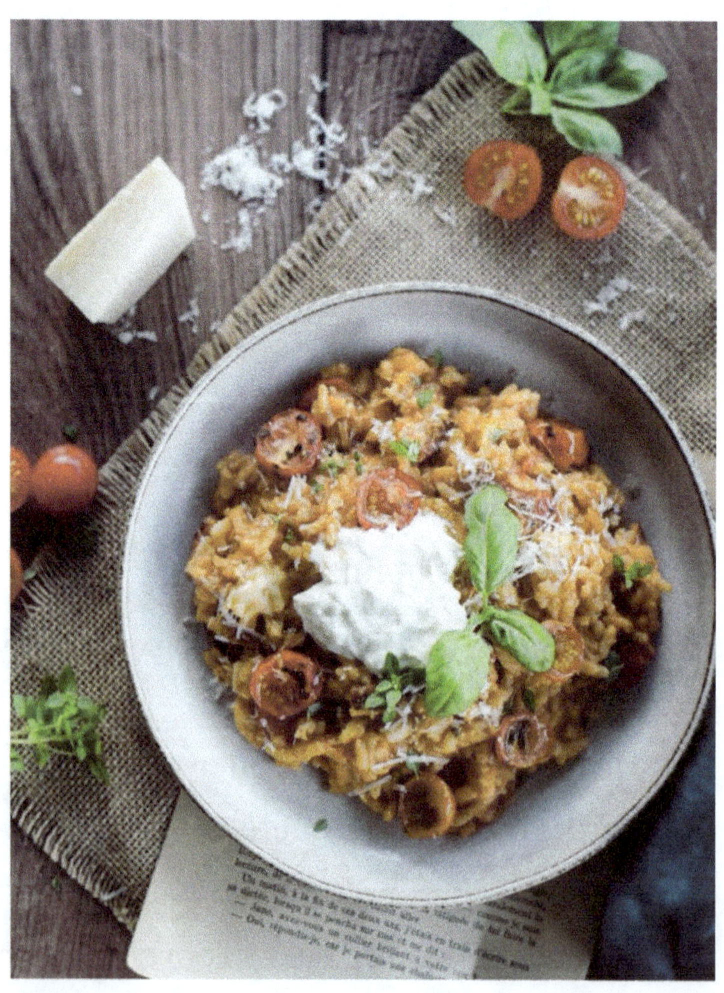

Oats Coffee Smoothie

Servings: 2

Cooking Time: 5 Minutes

Ingredients:

- 1 cup Oats, uncooked & grounded
- 2 tbsp. Instant Coffee
- 3 cup Milk, skimmed
- 2 Banana, frozen & sliced into chunks
- 2 tbsp. Flax Seeds, grounded

Directions:

1. Place all of the ingredients in a high-speed blender and blend for 2 minutes or until smooth and luscious.
2. Serve and enjoy.

Nutrition Info: Calories: 251Kcal; Carbs 10.9g; Proteins: 20.3g; Fat: 15.1g; Sodium: 102mg

Premium Roasted Baby Potatoes

Servings: 4

Cooking Time: 35 Minutes

Ingredients:

- 2 pounds' new yellow potatoes, scrubbed and cut into wedges
- 2 tablespoons extra virgin olive oil
- 2 teaspoons fresh rosemary, chopped
- 1 teaspoon garlic powder
- 1 teaspoon sweet paprika
- ½ teaspoon sea salt
- ½ teaspoon freshly ground black pepper

Directions:

1. Pre-heat your oven to 400 degrees Fahrenheit.
2. Line baking sheet with aluminum foil and set it aside.
3. Take a large bowl and add potatoes, olive oil, garlic, rosemary, paprika, sea salt and pepper.

4. Spread potatoes in single layer on baking sheet and bake for 35 minutes.

5. Serve and enjoy!

Nutrition Info: Calories: 225 Fat: 7g Carbohydrates: 37g Protein: 5g

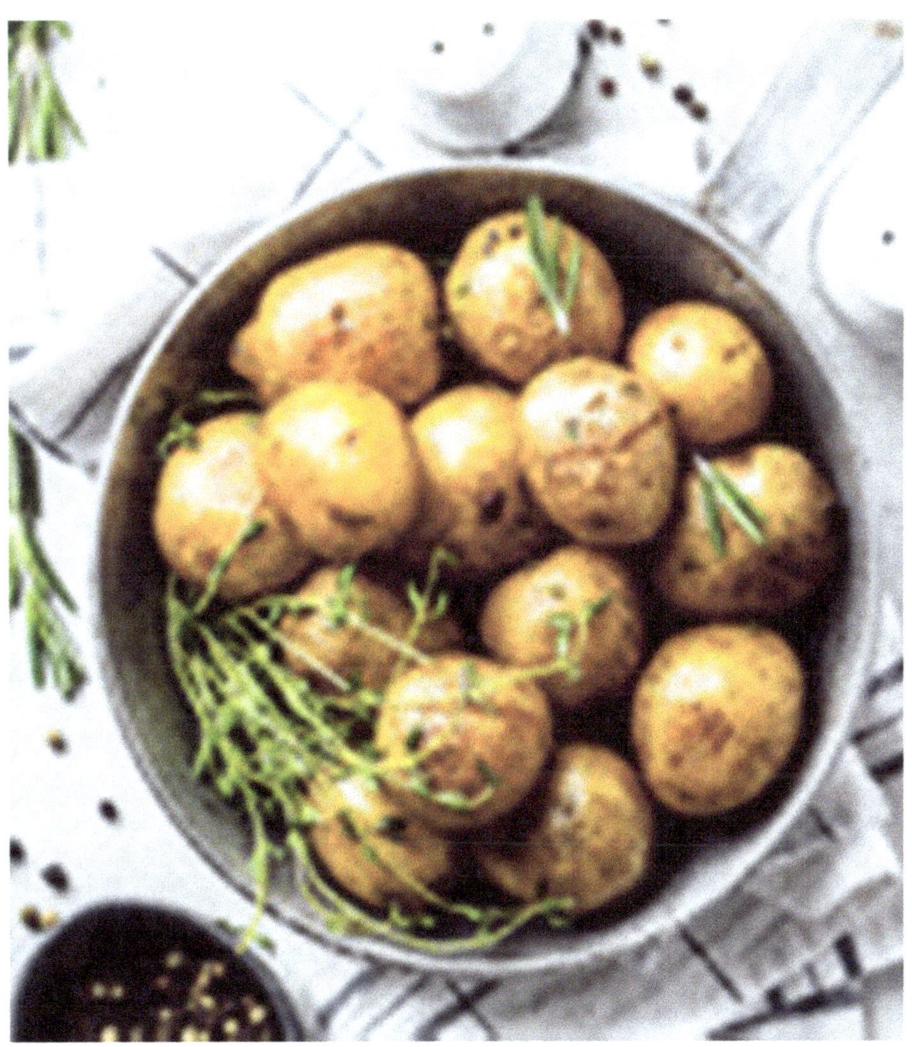

Chicken, Strawberry, And Avocado Salad

Cooking Time: 5 Minutes

Ingredients:

- 1,5 cups chicken (skin removed)
- 1/4 cup almonds
- 2 (5-oz) pkg salad greens
- 1 (16-oz) pkg strawberries
- 1 avocado
- 1/4 cup green onion
- 1/4 cup lime juice
- 3 tbsp. extra virgin olive oil
- 2 tbsp. honey
- 1/4 tsp. salt
- 1/4 tsp. pepper

Directions:

1. Toast almonds until golden and fragrant.
2. Mix lime juice, oil, honey, salt, and pepper.

3. Mix greens, sliced strawberries, chicken, diced avocado, and sliced green onion and sliced almonds; drizzle with dressing. Toss to coat.

4. Yummy!

Nutrition Info: Calories 150 / Protein 15 g / Fat 10 g / Carbs 5 g

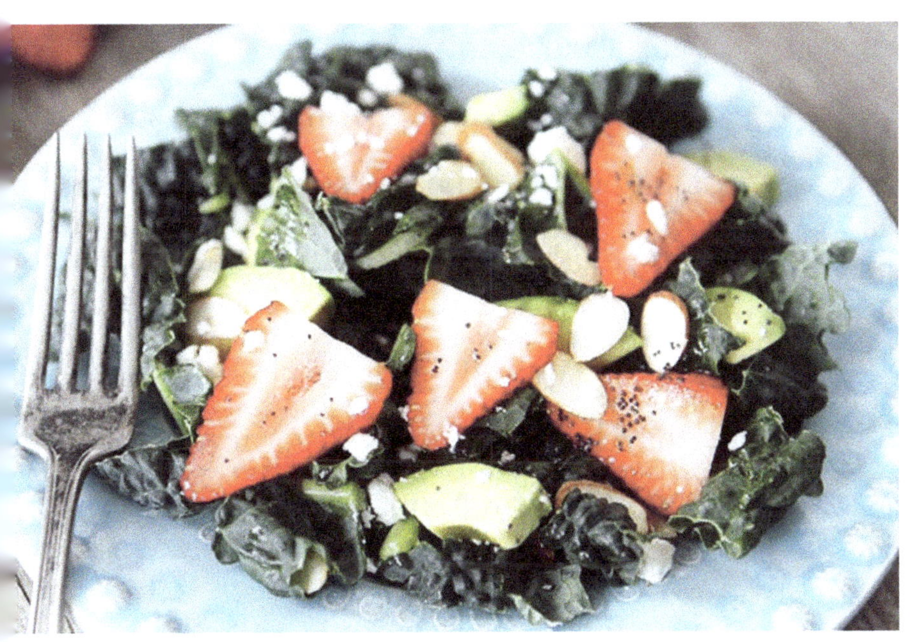

Lemony Brussels Sprout

Servings: 2

Cooking Time: 7 Minutes

Ingredients:

- ½ pound Brussels sprouts, halved
- 1 tablespoon olive oil
- 1 garlic clove, minced
- ½ teaspoon red pepper flakes, crushed
- Salt and ground black pepper, as required
- 1 tablespoon fresh lemon juice

Directions:

1. Heat the olive oil in a large skillet over medium heat and cook the garlic and red pepper flakes for about 1 minute, stirring continuously.
2. Stir in the Brussels sprouts, salt and black pepper and sauté for about 4-5 minutes.
3. Stir in lemon juice and sauté for about 1 minute more.

4. Serve hot.

5. Meal Prep Tip: Transfer the Brussels sprouts into a large bowl and set aside to cool completely. Divide the Brussels sprouts into 2 containers evenly. Cover the containers and refrigerate for about 1-2 days. Reheat in the microwave before serving.

Nutrition Info: Calories 114 Total Fat 7.5 g Saturated Fat 1.2 g Cholesterol 0 mg Total Carbs 11.2 g Sugar 2.7 g Fiber 4.4 g Sodium 108 mg Potassium 465 mg Protein 4.1 g

Easy Egg Salad

Servings: 4

Cooking Time: 15 To 20 Minutes

Ingredients:

- 6 Eggs, preferably free-range
- ¼ tsp. Salt
- 2 tbsp. Mayonnaise
- 1 tsp. Lemon juice
- 1 tsp. Dijon mustard
- Pepper, to taste
- Lettuce leaves, to serve

Directions:

1. Keep the eggs in a saucepan of water and pour cold water until it covers the egg by another 1 inch.
2. Bring to a boil and then remove the eggs from heat.
3. Peel the eggs under cold running water.

4. Transfer the cooked eggs into a food processor and pulse them until chopped.

5. Stir in the mayonnaise, lemon juice, salt, Dijon mustard, and pepper and mix them well.

6. Taste for seasoning and add more if required.

7. Serve in the lettuce leaves.

Nutrition Info: Calories – 166kcal; Fat – 14g; Carbohydrates - 0.85g; Proteins – 10g; Sodium: 132mg

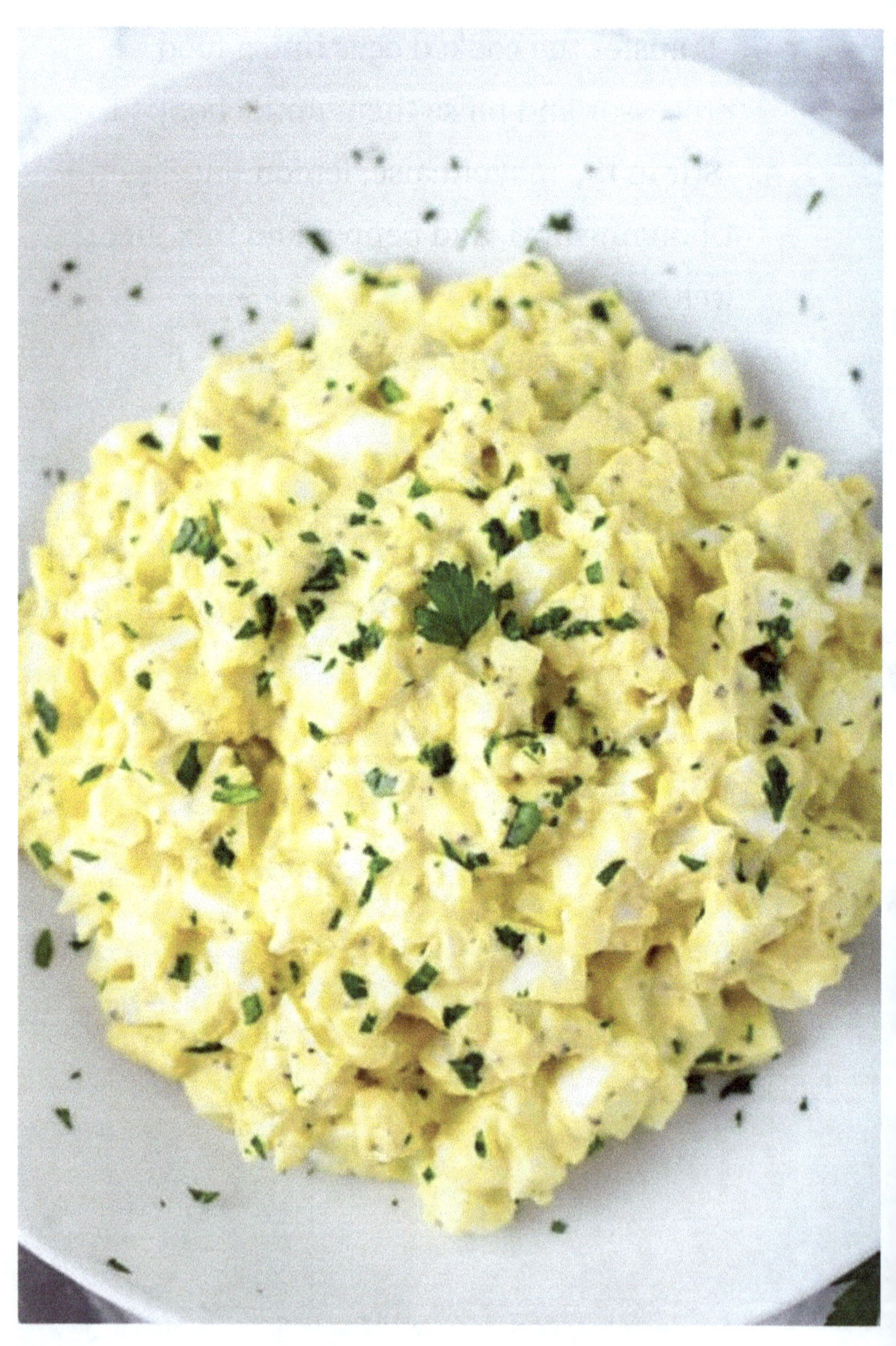

Cherry Tomato Salad

Servings: 6

Cooking Time: None

Ingredients:

- 40 cherry tomatoes, halved
- 1 cup mozzarella balls, halved
- 1 cup green olives, sliced
- 1 can (6 oz) black olives, sliced
- 2 green onions, chopped
- 3 oz roasted pine nuts
- Dressing:
- ½ cup olive oil
- 2 tbsp red wine vinegar
- 1 tsp dried oregano
- Salt and pepper to taste

Directions:

1. In a salad bowl, combine the tomatoes, olives and onions.
2. Prepare the dressing by combining olive oil with red wine vinegar, dried oregano, salt and pepper.
3. Sprinkle with the dressing and add the nuts.
4. Let marinate in the fridge for 1 hour.

Nutrition Info: Carbohydrates: 10.7 g Protein: 2.4 g Total sugars: 3.6 g

Spaghetti Squash Mash

Servings: 4

Cooking Time: 1 Hour

Ingredients:

- Spaghetti squash (halved, seeds removed) - 1
- Olive oil: 2 tablespoon
- Garlic powder: 1 teaspoon
- Dried rosemary: 1 teaspoon
- Dried parsley: 1 teaspoon
- Dried thyme: 1 teaspoon
- Sage: ½ teaspoon
- Salt: 1 teaspoon
- Cracked pepper: ½ teaspoon

Directions:

1.   Put a little water in a baking pan and place the squash halves in it, cut side down.
2.   Roast in an oven preheated to 350 degrees Fahrenheit for 45 minutes to an hour.
3.   Remove, leave to cool and then scoop out all the flesh.
4.   Place the squash in a bowl and mix in the rest of the ingredients.
5.   Place in the oven and cook for 15 minutes more.

Nutrition Info: 91 Cal, 7 g total fat, 5.5 g net carb., 1.5 g fiber, 3 g protein.

Quick Zucchini Bowl

Servings: 4

Cooking Time: 10 Minutes

Ingredients:

- ½ pound of pasta
- 2 tablespoons of olive oil
- 6 crushed garlic cloves
- 1 teaspoon of red chili
- 2 finely sliced spring onions
- 3 teaspoons of chopped rosemary
- 1 large zucchini cut up in half, lengthways and sliced
- 5 large portabella mushrooms
- 1 can of tomatoes
- 4 tablespoons of Parmesan cheese
- Fresh ground black pepper

Directions:

1. Cook the pasta in boiling water until Al Dente.
2. Take a large-sized frying pan and place over medium heat.
3. Add oil and allow the oil to heat up.
4. Add garlic, onion and chili and sauté for a few minutes until golden.
5. Add zucchini, rosemary and mushroom and sauté for a few minutes.
6. Increase the heat to medium-high and add tinned tomatoes to the sauce until thick.
7. Drain your boiled pasta and transfer to a serving platter.
8. Pour the tomato mix on top and mix using tongs.
9. Garnish with Parmesan cheese and freshly ground black pepper.
10. Enjoy!

Nutrition Info: Calories: 361 Fat: 12g Carbohydrates: 47g Protein: 14g

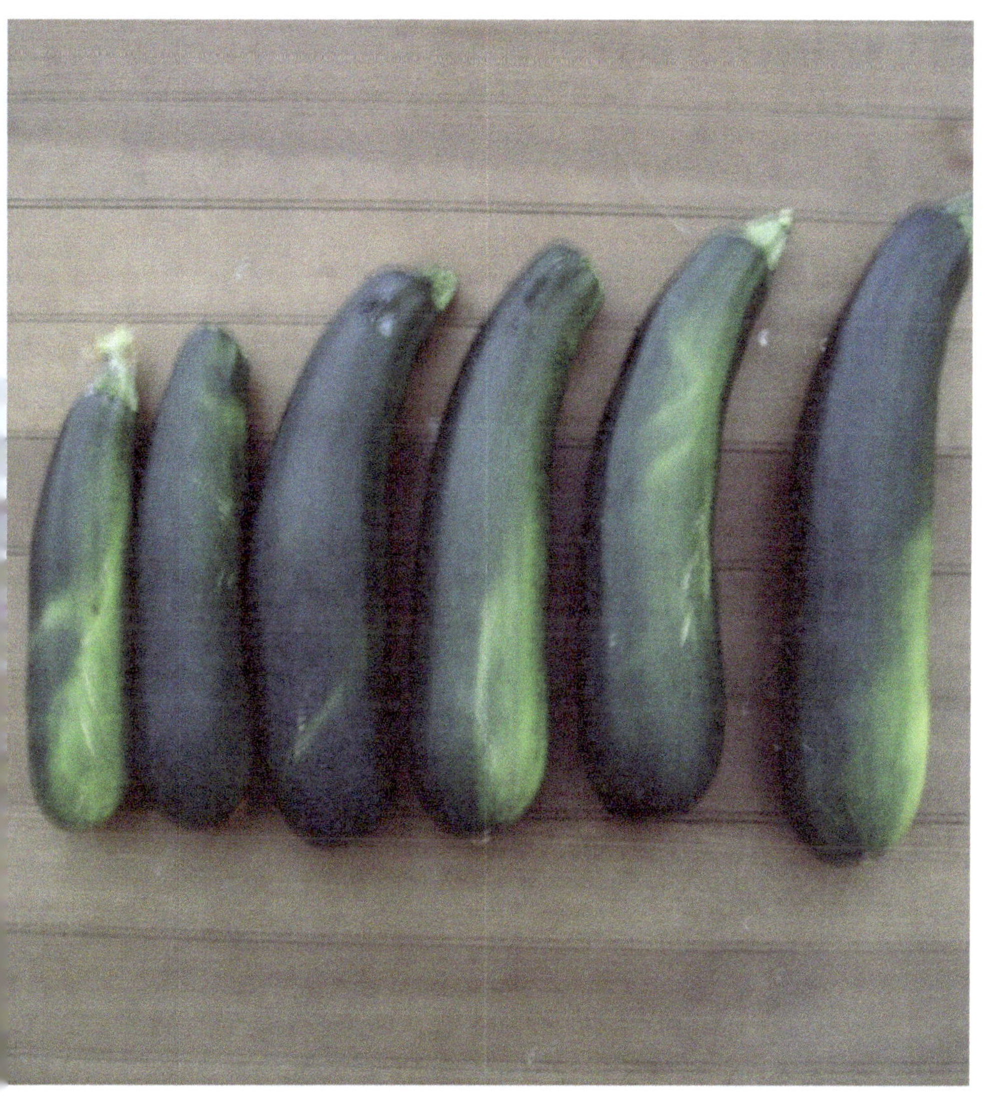

Blueberry Smoothie

Servings: 2

Cooking Time: 2 Minutes

Ingredients:

- 1 tbsp. Lemon Juice
- 1 ¾ cup Coconut Milk, full-fat
- 1/2 tsp. Vanilla Extract
- 3 oz. Blueberries, frozen

Directions:

1. Combine coconut milk, blueberries, lemon juice, and vanilla extract in a high-speed blender.
2. Blend for 2 minutes for a smooth and luscious smoothie.
3. Serve and enjoy.

Nutrition Info: Calories: 417cal; Carbohydrates: 9g; Proteins: 4g; Fat: 43g; Sodium: 35mg

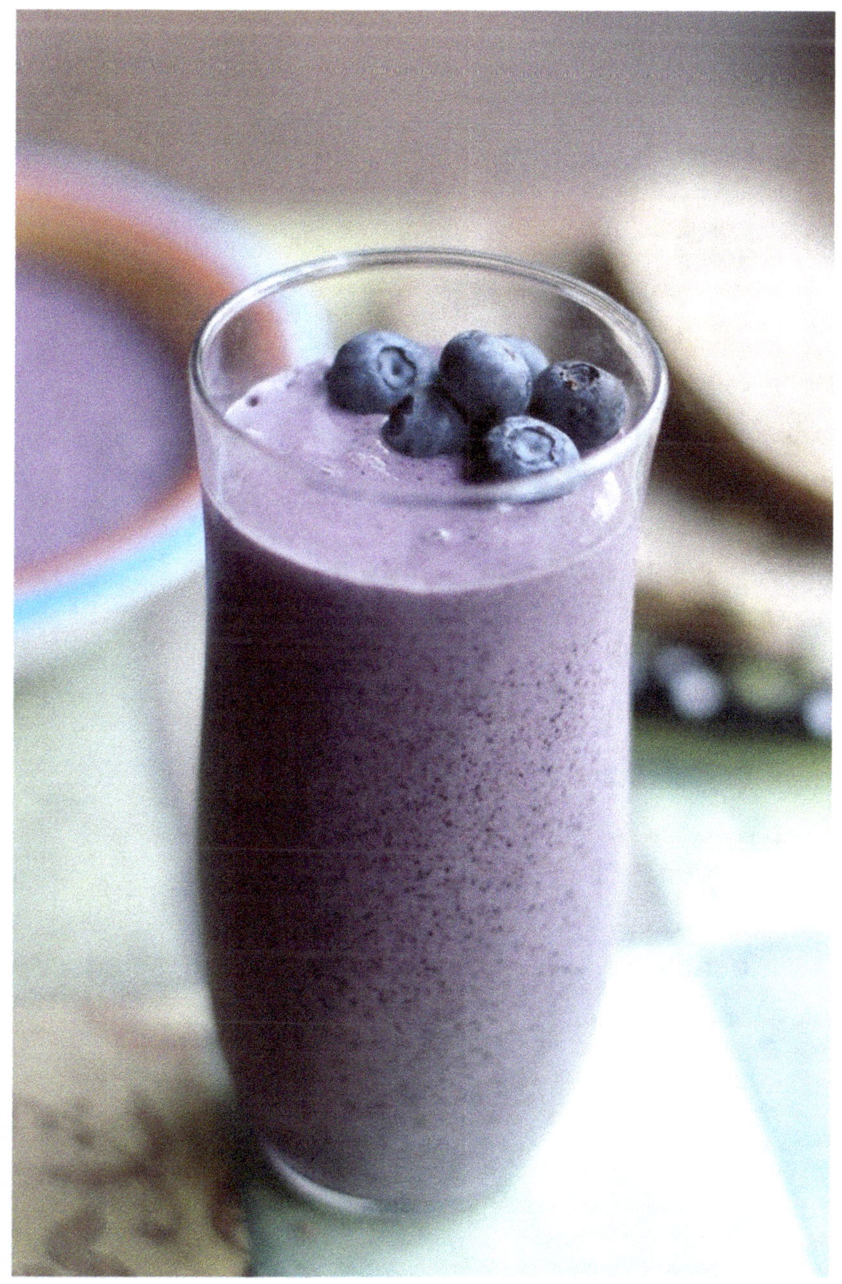

Beef Chili

Servings: 4

Cooking Time: 20 Minutes

Ingredients:

- 1/2 tsp. Garlic Powder
- 1 tsp. Coriander, grounded
- 1 lb. Beef, grounded
- 1/2 tsp. Sea Salt
- 1/2 tsp. Cayenne Pepper
- 1 tsp. Cumin, grounded
- 1/2 tsp. Pepper, grounded
- 1/2 cup Salsa, low-carb & no-sugar

Directions:

1. Heat a large-sized pan over medium-high heat and cook the beef in it until browned.
2. Stir in all the spices and cook them for 7 minutes or until everything is combined.
3. When the beef gets cooked, spoon in the salsa.

4.   Bring the mixture to a simmer and cook for another 8 minutes or until everything comes together.

5.   Take it from heat and transfer to a serving bowl.

Nutrition Info: Calories: 229Kcal; Fat: 10g; Carbohydrates: 2g; Proteins: 33g; Sodium: 675mg

Avocado Turmeric Smoothie

Servings: 1

Cooking Time: 2 Minutes

Ingredients:

- 1/2 of 1 Avocado
- 1 cup Ice, crushed
- ¾ cup Coconut Milk, full-fat
- 1 tsp. Lemon Juice
- ¼ cup Almond Milk
- 1/2 tsp. Turmeric
- 1 tsp. Ginger, freshly grated

Directions:

1. Place all the ingredients excluding the crushed ice in a high-speed blender and blend for 2 to 3 minutes or until smooth.
2. Transfer to a serving glass and enjoy it.

Nutrition Info: Calories: 232cal; Carbs: 4.1g; Proteins: 1.7g; Fat: 22.4g; Sodium: 25mg

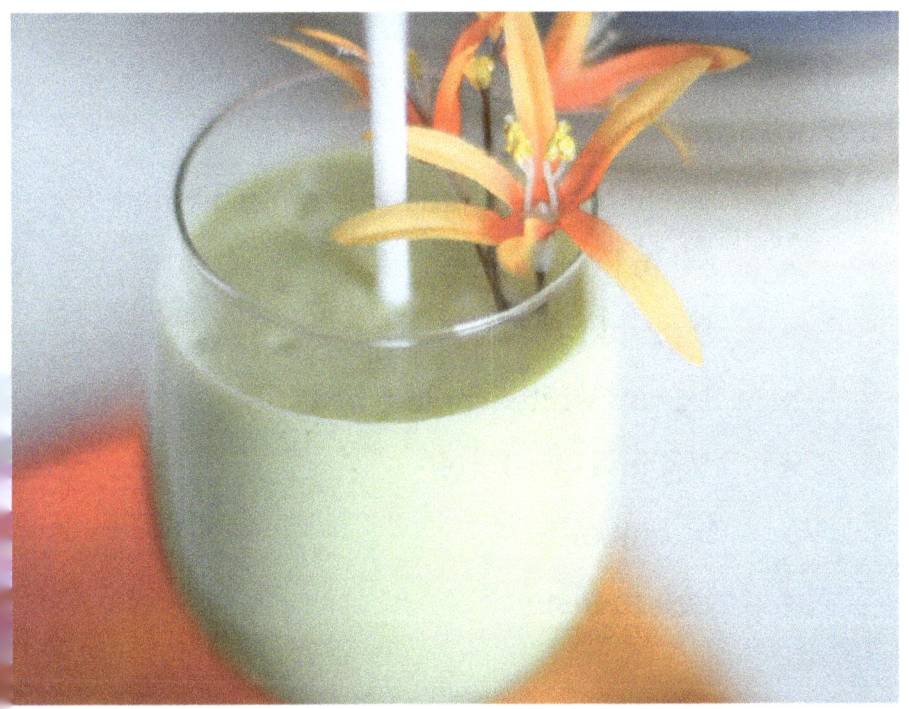

Fried Okra

Servings: 4

Cooking Time: 15 Minutes

Ingredients:

- 2 teaspoons Cajun seasoning, divided
- 1 cup buttermilk
- 8 oz. okra
- ½ cup white whole-wheat flour
- ½ cup cornstarch
- ⅓ cup oil
- Salt to taste

Directions:

1. Mix half of the Cajun seasoning and buttermilk in a bowl.
2. Add the okra.
3. Mix well.
4. Let sit for 10 minutes.

5. In another bowl, blend the remaining Cajun seasoning, flour and cornstarch.

6. Drain the okra.

7. Dip each okra in the flour mixture.

8. Pour the oil in a pan over medium high heat.

9. Cook the okra until golden on all sides.

10. Season with salt before serving.

Nutrition Info: Calories 106 Total Fat 5 g Saturated Fat 0 g Cholesterol 0 mg Sodium 75 mg Total Carbohydrate 14 g Dietary Fiber 2 g Total Sugars 1 g Protein 2 g Potassium 195 mg

Cinnamon Roll Smoothie

Servings: 1

Cooking Time: 0 Minutes

Ingredients:

- 1 tsp. Flax Meal or oats, if preferred
- 1 cup Almond Milk
- 1/2 tsp. Cinnamon
- 2 tbsp. Protein Powder
- 1 cup Ice
- ¼ tsp. Vanilla Extract
- 4 tsp. Sweetener of your choice

Directions:

1. Pour the milk into the blender, followed by the protein powder, sweetener, flax meal, cinnamon, vanilla extract, and ice.
2. Blend for 40 seconds or until smooth.
3. Serve and enjoy.

Nutrition Info: Calories: 145cal; Carbs: 1.6g; Proteins: 26.5g; Fat: 3.25g; Sodium: 30mg

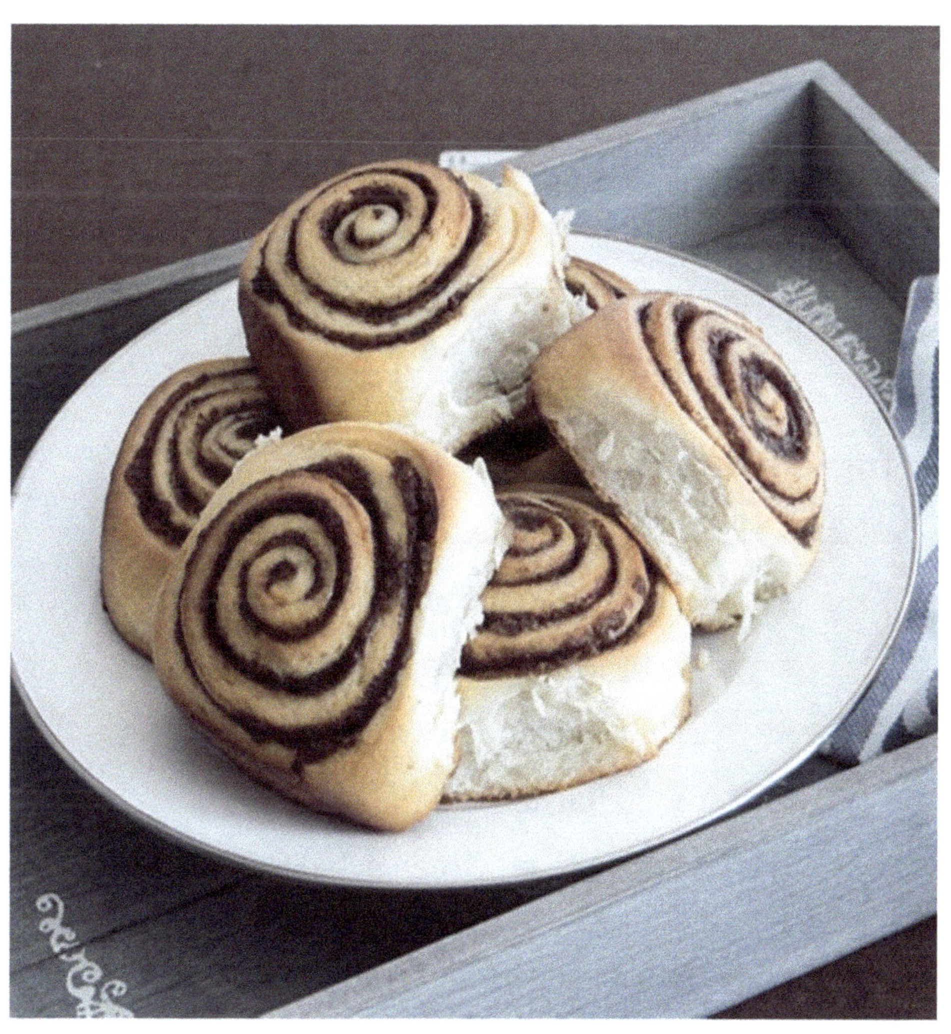

Cobb Salad

Servings: 1

Cooking Time: 5 Minutes

Ingredients:

- 4 Cherry Tomatoes, chopped
- ¼ cup Bacon, cooked & crumbled
- 1/2 of 1 Avocado, chopped
- 2 oz. Chicken Breast, shredded
- 1 Egg, hardboiled
- 2 cups Mixed Green salad
- 1 oz. Feta Cheese, crumbled

Directions:

1. Toss all the ingredients for the Cobb salad in a large mixing bowl and toss well.
2. Serve and enjoy it.

Nutrition Info: Calories: 307Kcal; Carbohydrates: 3g; Proteins: 27g; Fat: 20g; Sodium: 522mg

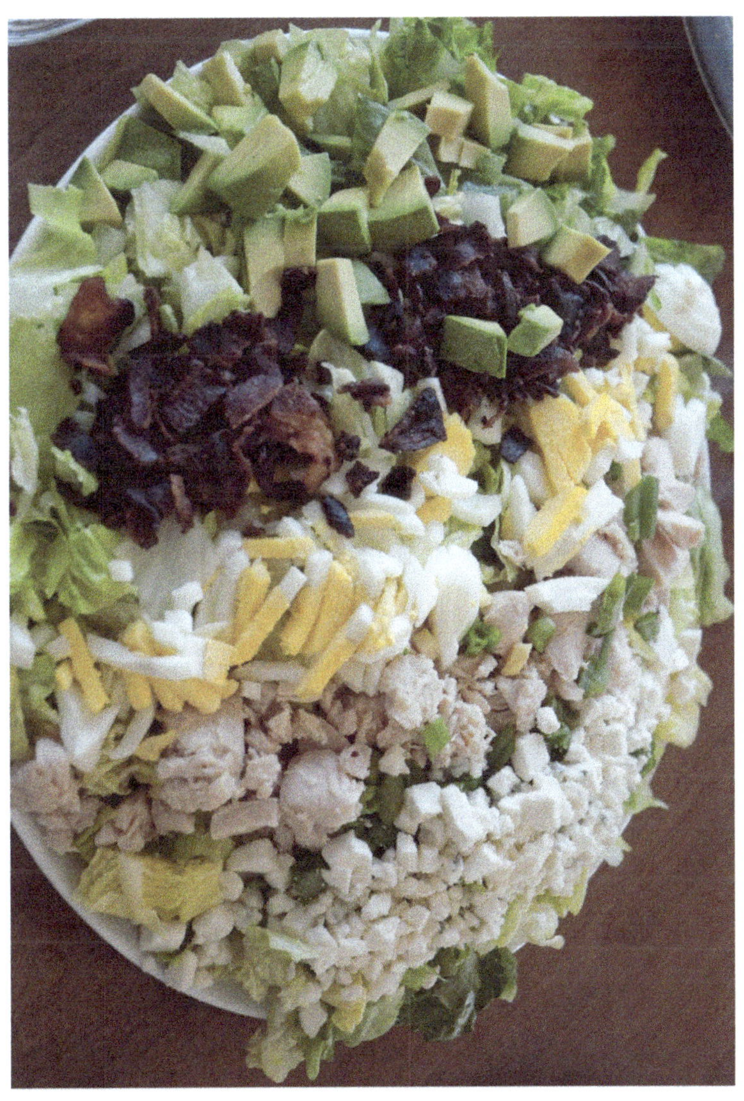

Garlic Sautée D Spinach

Servings: 4

Cooking Time: 10 Minutes

Ingredients:

- 1 1/2 tablespoons olive oil
- 4 cloves minced garlic
- 6 cups fresh baby spinach
- Salt and pepper

Directions:

1. Heat the oil in a large skillet over medium-high heat.
2. Add the garlic and cook for 1 minute.
3. Stir in the spinach and season with salt and pepper.
4. Sauté for 1 to 2 minutes until just wilted. Serve hot.

Nutrition Info: Calories 60, Total Fat 5.5g, Saturated Fat 0.8g, Total Carbs 2.6g, Net Carbs 1.5g, Protein 1.5g, Sugar 0.2g, Fiber 1.1g, Sodium 36mg

Garlic Bread

Servings: 4-5

Cooking Time: 15 Minutes

Ingredients:

- 2 stale French rolls
- 4 tbsp. crushed or crumpled garlic
- 1 cup of mayonnaise
- Powdered grated Parmesan
- 1 tbsp. olive oil

Directions:

1. Preheat the air fryer. Set the time of 5 minutes and the temperature to 2000C.
2. Mix mayonnaise with garlic and set aside.
3. Cut the baguettes into slices, but without separating them completely.
4. Fill the cavities of equals. Brush with olive oil and sprinkle with grated cheese.

5. Place in the basket of the air fryer. Set the timer to 10 minutes, adjust the temperature to 1800C and press the power button.

Nutrition Info: Calories: 340 Fat: 15g Carbohydrates: 32g Protein: 15g Sugar: 0g Cholesterol: 0mg

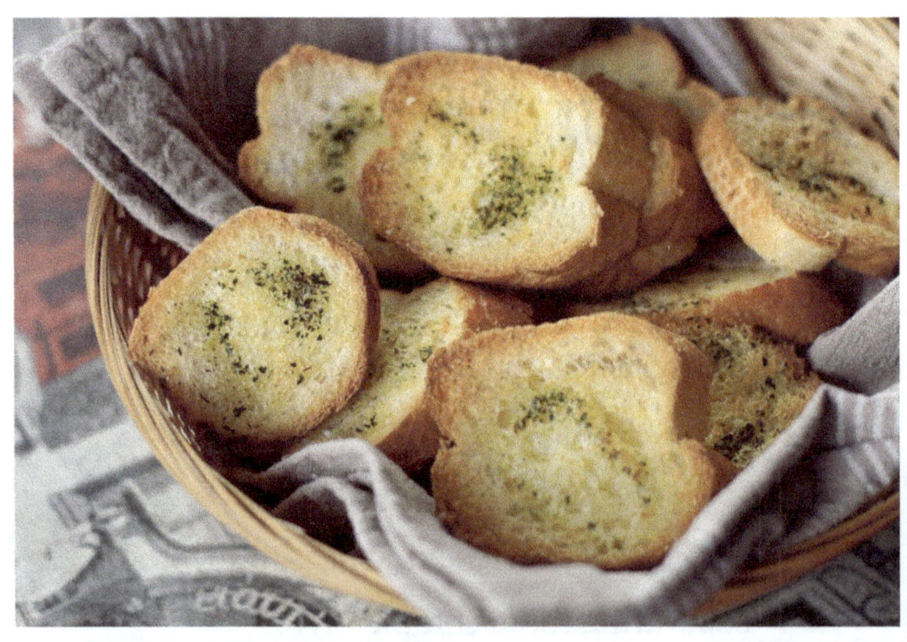

Tuna Avocado Salad

Servings: 4

Cooking Time: 0 Minutes

Ingredients:

- 1 avocado, pit removed and sliced
- 1 lemon, juiced
- 1 tablespoon chopped onion
- 5 ounces cooked or canned tuna
- Salt and pepper to taste

Directions:

1. In a mixing bowl, combine the avocado and lime juice. Mash the avocado and add the tuna.
2. Season with salt and pepper to taste.
3. Serve chilled.

Nutrition Info: Calories: 695.5g Fat: 50.7 g Protein: 41.5 g Carbs: 18.3 g

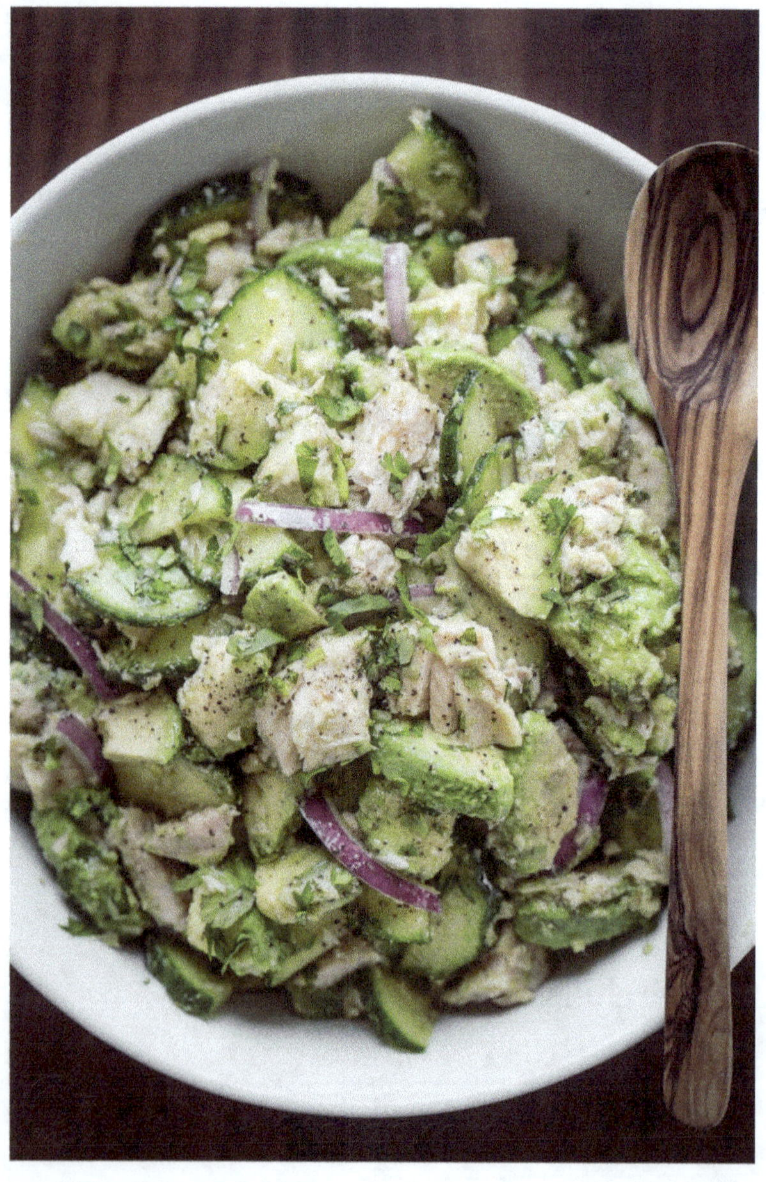

French Toast In Sticks

Servings: 4

Cooking Time: 10 Minutes

Ingredients:

- 4 slices of white bread, 38 mm thick, preferably hard
- 2 eggs
- 60 ml of milk
- 15 ml maple sauce
- 2 ml vanilla extract
- Nonstick Spray Oil
- 38g of sugar
- 3ground cinnamon
- Maple syrup, to serve
- Sugar to sprinkle

Directions:

1. Cut each slice of bread into thirds making 12 pieces. Place sideways
2. Beat the eggs, milk, maple syrup and vanilla.

3. Preheat the air fryer, set it to 175C.

4. Dip the sliced bread in the egg mixture and place it in the preheated air fryer. Sprinkle French toast generously with oil spray.

5. Cook French toast for 10 minutes at 175C. Turn the toast halfway through cooking.

6. Mix the sugar and cinnamon in a bowl.

7. Cover the French toast with the sugar and cinnamon mixture when you have finished cooking.

8. Serve with Maple syrup and sprinkle with powdered sugar

Nutrition Info: Calories 128 Fat 6.2 g, Carbohydrates 16.3 g, Sugar 3.3 g, Protein 3.2 g, Cholesterol 17 mg

Strawberry Salsa

Servings: 4

Cooking Time: 5 Minutes;

Ingredients:

- 4 tomatoes, seeded and chopped
- 1-pint strawberry, chopped
- 1 red onion, chopped
- 2 tablespoons of juice from a lime
- 1 jalapeno pepper, minced
- What you will need from the store cupboard:
- 1 tablespoon olive oil
- 2 garlic cloves, minced

Directions:

1. Bring together the strawberries, tomatoes, jalapeno, and onion in the bowl.
2. Stir in the garlic, oil, and lime juice.
3. Refrigerate. Serve with separately cooked pork or poultry.

Nutrition Info: Calories 19, Carbs 3g, Fiber 1g, Sugar 0.2g, Cholesterol 0mg, Total Fat 1g, Protein 0g

45

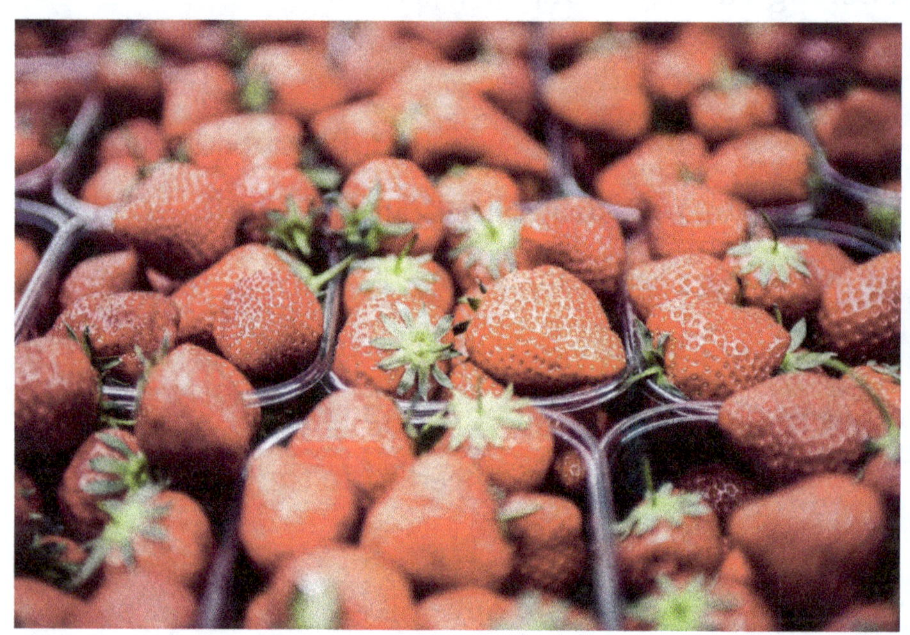

Southwestern Bean-and-pepper Salad

Servings: 4

Cooking Time: 0 Minutes

Ingredients:

- 1 (15-ounce) can pinto beans, drained and rinsed
- 2 bell peppers, cored and chopped
- 1 cup corn kernels (cut from 1 to 2 ears or frozen and thawed)
- Salt
- Freshly ground black pepper
- Juice of 2 limes
- 1 tablespoon olive oil
- 1 avocado, chopped

Directions:

1. In a large bowl, combine beans, peppers, corn, salt, and pepper. Squeeze fresh lime juice to taste and stir in olive oil. Let the mixture stand in the refrigerator for 30 minutes.

2. Add avocado just before serving.

3. Budget-saver tip avocado prices can vary dramatically depending on their availability. In addition, while avocado in your salad can really add flavor and satiety, for an equally delicious salad you could add a cup of cooked and chopped sweet potatoes with 1 to 2 tablespoons of sunflower seeds.

Nutrition Info: Total calories: 245 Total fat: 11g Saturated fat: 2g Cholesterol: 0mg Sodium: 97mg Potassium: 380mg Total carbohydrate: 32g Fiber: 10g Sugars: 4g Protein: 8g.

Sautéed Turkey Bowl

Servings: 1

Cooking Time: 10 Minutes

Ingredients:

- 4 ounces boneless, skinless turkey breast
- 1 teaspoon olive oil
- 1 ½ teaspoons balsamic vinegar
- ½ teaspoon dried basil
- ¼ teaspoon dried thyme
- Salt and pepper
- ¼ cup instant brown rice

Directions:

1. Toss the turkey with the olive oil, balsamic vinegar, basil, and thyme.
2. Season lightly with salt and pepper then cover and chill for 20 minutes.
3. Bring ¼ cup of water to boil in a small saucepan.

4. Stir in the brown rice then simmer for 5 minutes and remove from heat, covered.

5. Meanwhile, heat a small skillet over medium heat and grease lightly with cooking spray.

6. Add the marinated turkey and sauté for 6 to 8 minutes until cooked through.

7. Spoon the turkey over the brown rice and serve hot.

Nutrition Info: Calories 200, Total Fat 6.8g, Saturated Fat 1.1g, Total Carbs 13.3g, Net Carbs 12.1g, Protein 20.4g, Sugar 4g, Fiber 1.2g, Sodium 1152mg

Cauliflower & Apple Salad

Servings: 4

Cooking Time: 0 Minutes

Ingredients:

- 3 Cups Cauliflower, Chopped into Florets
- 2 Cups Baby Kale
- 1 Sweet Apple, Cored & Chopped
- ¼ Cup Basil, Fresh & Chopped
- ¼ Cup Mint, Fresh & Chopped
- ¼ Cup Parsley, Fresh & Chopped
- 1/3 Cup Scallions, Sliced Thin
- 2 Tablespoons Yellow Raisins
- 1 Tablespoon Sun Dried Tomatoes, Chopped
- ½ Cup Miso Dressing, Optional
- ¼ Cup Roasted Pumpkin Seeds, Optional

Directions:

1. Combine everything together, tossing before serving.

2. Interesting Facts: This vegetable is an extremely high source of vitamin A, vitamin B1, B2 and B3.

Nutrition Info: Calories: 198 Protein: 7 Grams Fat: 8 Grams Carbs: 32 Grams

Zucchini Risotto

Servings: 4

Cooking Time: 30 Minutes

Ingredients:

- ½ cup shallots, chopped
- tablespoons olive oil
- garlic cloves, minced
- cups cauliflower rice
- cup zucchinis, cubed
- cups veggie stock
- ½ cup white mushrooms, chopped
- ½ teaspoon coriander, ground
- A pinch of salt and black pepper
- ¼ teaspoon oregano, dried
- tablespoons parsley, chopped

Directions:

1. Heat up a pan with the oil over medium heat, add the shallots, garlic, mushrooms,

coriander and oregano, stir and sauté for 10
minutes.

2.   Add the cauliflower rice and the other
    ingredients, toss, cook for 20 minutes more,
    divide between plates and serve.

Nutrition Info: Calories 231 fat 5 fiber 3 carbs 9
protein 12

Peanut Butter Mousse

Servings: 2

Cooking Time: 10 Minutes

Ingredients:

- 1 tbsp. peanut butter
- 1 tsp. vanilla extract
- 1 tsp. stevia
- 1/2 cup heavy cream

Directions:

1. Add all ingredients into the bowl and whisk until soft peak forms.
2. Spoon into the serving bowls and enjoy.

Nutrition Info: Calories 157 Fat 15.1 g, Carbohydrates 5.2 g, Sugar 3.6 g, Protein 2.6 g, Cholesterol 41 mg

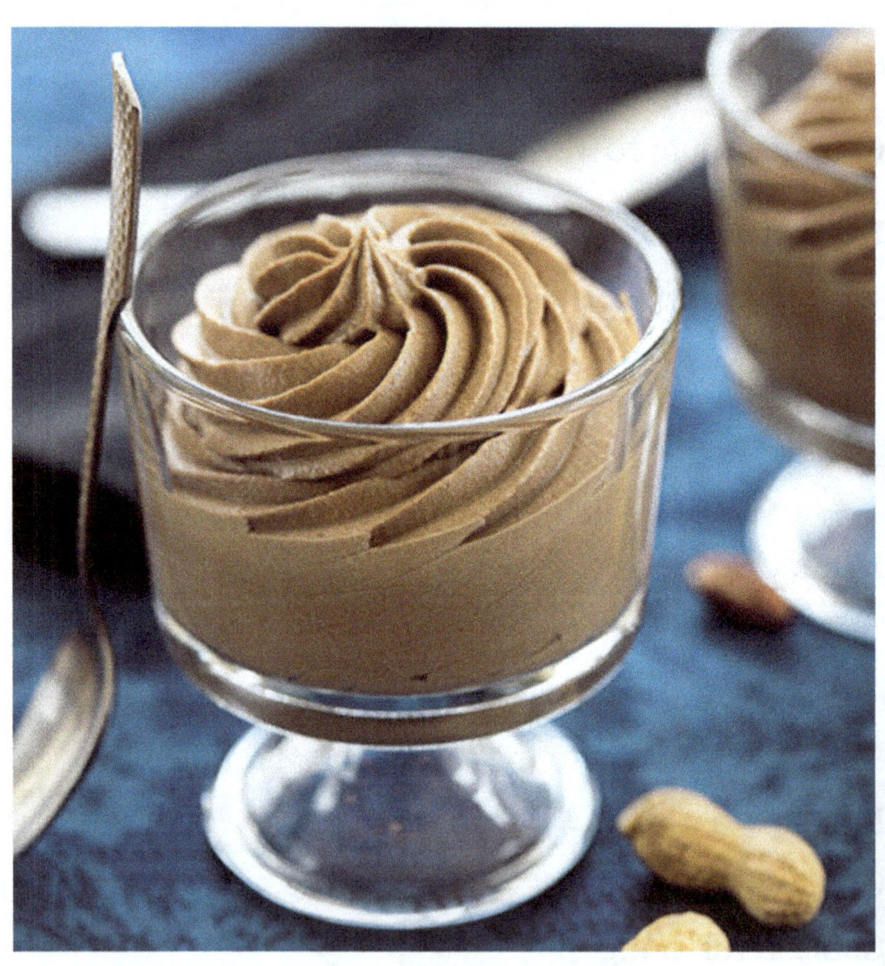

Peanut Butter Banana Smoothie

Servings: 1

Cooking Time: 2 Minutes

Ingredients:

- ¼ cup Greek Yoghurt, plain
- 1/2 tbsp. Chia Seeds
- 1/2 cup Ice Cubes
- 1/2 of 1 Banana
- 1/2 cup Water
- 1 tbsp. Peanut Butter

Directions:

1. Place all the ingredients needed to make the smoothie in a high-speed blender and blend to get a smooth and luscious mixture.
2. Transfer the smoothie to a serving glass and enjoy it.

Nutrition Info: Calories: 202cal; Carbohydrates: 14g; Proteins: 10g; Fat: 9g; Sodium: 30mg

Salmon With Asparagus

Servings: 3

Cooking Time: 10 Minutes

Ingredients:

- 1 lb. Salmon, sliced into fillets

- 1 tbsp. Olive Oil

- Salt & Pepper, as needed

- 1 bunch of Asparagus, trimmed

- 2 cloves of Garlic, minced

- Zest & Juice of 1/2 Lemon

- 1 tbsp. Butter, salted

Directions:

1. Spoon in the butter and olive oil into a large pan and heat it over medium-high heat.

2. Once it becomes hot, place the salmon and season it with salt and pepper.

3. Cook for 4 minutes per side and then cook the other side.

4. Stir in the garlic and lemon zest to it.

5. Cook for further 2 minutes or until slightly browned.

6. Off the heat and squeeze the lemon juice over it.

7. Serve it hot.

Nutrition Info: Calories: 409Kcal; Carbohydrates: 2.7g; Proteins: 32.8g; Fat: 28.8g; Sodium: 497mg

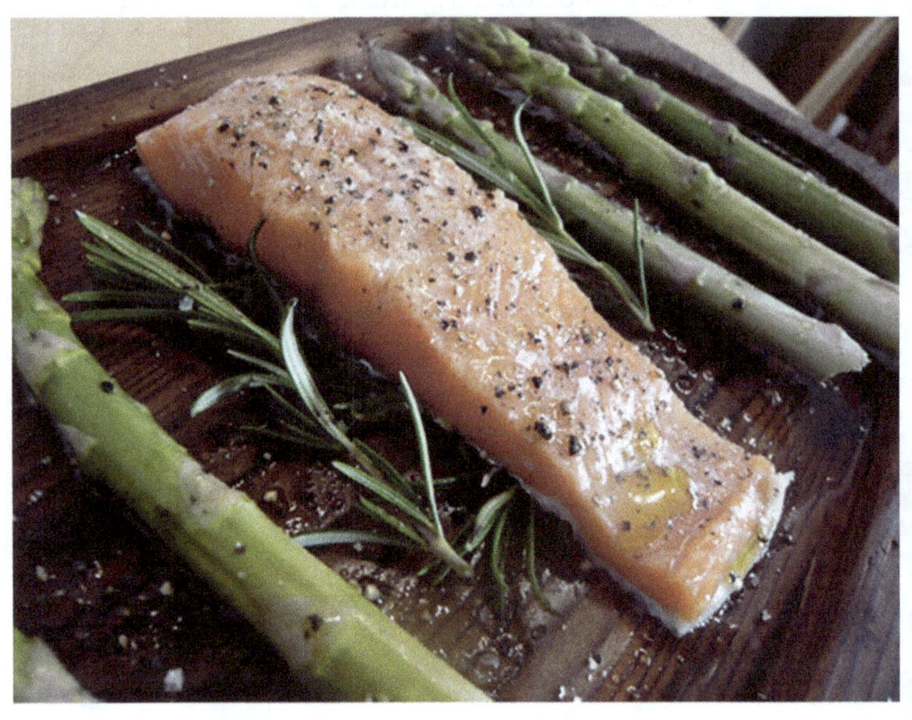

Roasted Tomatoes

Servings: 4

Cooking Time: 25 Minutes

Ingredients:

- 1-pound tomatoes, halved
- A pinch of salt and black pepper
- 2 tablespoons olive oil
- 1 teaspoon rosemary, dried
- 1 teaspoon basil, dried
- 1 tablespoon chives, chopped

Directions:

1. In a roasting pan combine the tomatoes with the oil and the other ingredients, toss gently and bake at 390 degrees F for 25 minutes.
2. Divide the mix between plates and serve.

Nutrition Info: calories 124 fat 14 fiber 4 carbs 4 protein 14

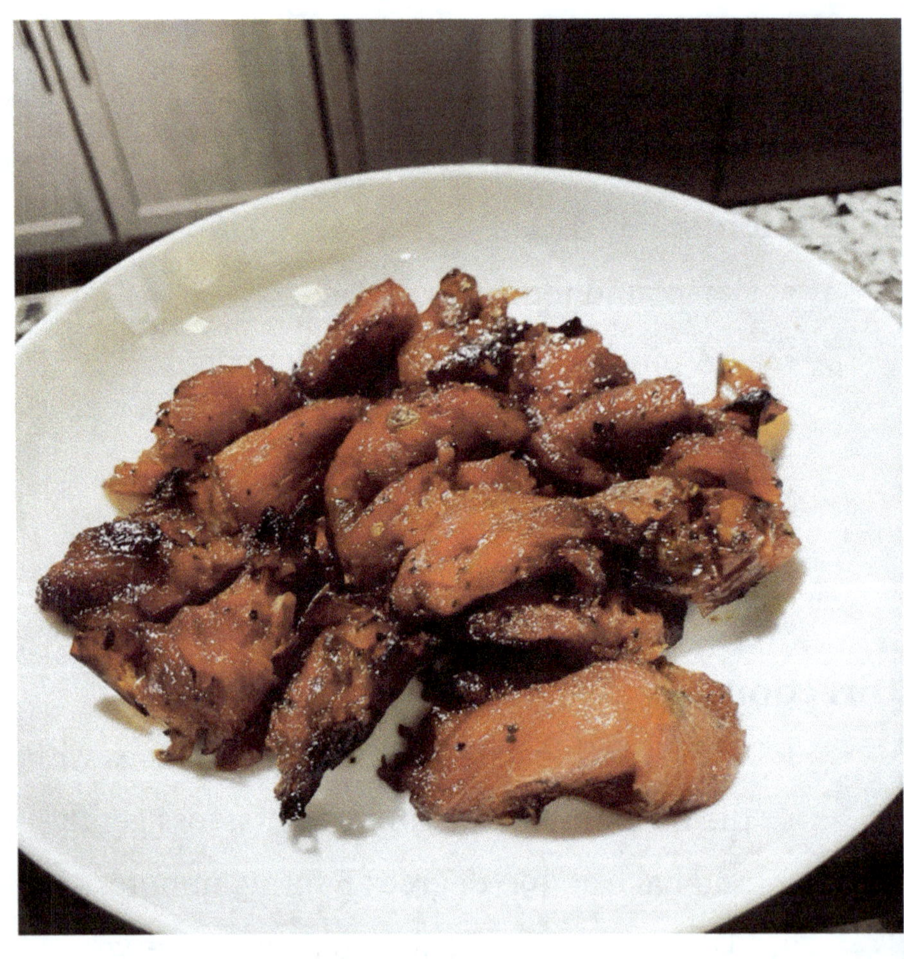

Crispy Radishes

Servings: 4

Cooking Time: 20 Minutes

Ingredients:

- Cooking spray
- 15 radishes, sliced
- Salt and black pepper to the taste
- 1 tablespoon chives, chopped

Directions:

1. Arrange radish slices on a lined baking sheet and spray them with cooking oil.
2. Season with salt and pepper and sprinkle chives, introduce in the oven at 375 degrees F and bake for 10 minutes.
3. Flip them and bake for 10 minutes more.
4. Serve them cold.
5. Enjoy!

Nutrition Info: calories 34 fat 4 fiber 0.4 carbs 4 protein 0.1

Edamame Salad

Servings: 1

Cooking Time: 0 Minutes

Ingredients:

- ¼ Cup Red Onion, Chopped
- 1 Cup Corn Kernels, Fresh
- 1 Cup Edamame Beans, Shelled & Thawed
- 1 Red Bell Pepper, Chopped
- 2-3 Tablespoons Lime Juice, Fresh
- 5-6 Basil Leaves, Fresh & Sliced
- 5-6 Mint Leaves, Fresh & Sliced
- Sea Salt & Black Pepper to Taste

Directions:

1. Place everything into a Mason jar, and then seal the jar tightly. Shake well before serving.

2. Interesting Facts: Whole corn is a fantastic source of phosphorus, magnesium, and B vitamins. It also promotes healthy digestion and contains heart-healthy antioxidants. It is

important to seek out organic corn in order to bypass all of the genetically modified product that is out on the market.

Nutrition Info: Calorics: 299 Protein: 20 Grams Fat: 9 Grams Carbs: 38 Grams

Summer Chickpea Salad

Servings: 4

Cooking Time: 15 Minutes

Ingredients:

- 1 ½ Cups Cherry Tomatoes, Halved
- 1 Cup English Cucumber, Slices
- 1 Cup Chickpeas, Canned, Unsalted, Drained & Rinsed
- ¼ Cup Red Onion, Slivered
- 2 Tablespoon Olive Oil
- 1 ½ Tablespoons Lemon Juice, Fresh
- 1 ½ Tablespoons Lemon Juice, Fresh
- Sea Salt & Black Pepper to Taste

Directions:

1. Mix everything together, and toss to combine before serving.

Nutrition Info: Calories: 145 Protein: 4 Grams Fat: 7.5 Grams Carbs: 16 Grams

Herbed Risotto

Servings: 4

Cooking Time: 25 Minutes

Ingredients:

- cups cauliflower rice
- scallions, chopped
- tablespoons avocado oil
- cups veggie stock
- Juice of 1 lime
- 1 tablespoon parsley, chopped
- 1 tablespoon cilantro, chopped
- 1 tablespoon basil, chopped
- 1 tablespoon oregano, chopped
- 1 teaspoon sweet paprika
- A pinch of salt and black pepper

Directions:

1. Heat up a pan with the oil over medium heat, add the scallions and sauté for 5 minutes.
2. Add the cauliflower rice, the stock and the other ingredients, toss, cook over medium heat for 20 minutes, divide between plates and serve as a side dish.

Nutrition Info: Calories 182 fat 4 fiber 2 carbs 8 protein 10

Roasted Radish With Fresh Herbs

Servings: 4

Cooking Time: 30 Minutes

Ingredients:

- 1 tbsp. coconut oil
- 1 bunch radishes
- 2 tbsps. Minced chives
- 1 tbsp. minced rosemary
- 1 tbsp. minced thyme

Directions:

1. Wash the radishes, then remove the tops and stems. Cut them into quarters and reserve.
2. Add the oil to a cast iron pan, then heat to medium. Add the radishes, then season with salt and pepper. Cook on medium heat for 6-8 minutes, until almost tender, then add the herbs and cook through.

3.   The radishes can be served warm with meats or chilled with salads.

Nutrition Info: Net carbs: 1.8g, Protein: .9g, Fat: 13g, Calories: 133kcal.

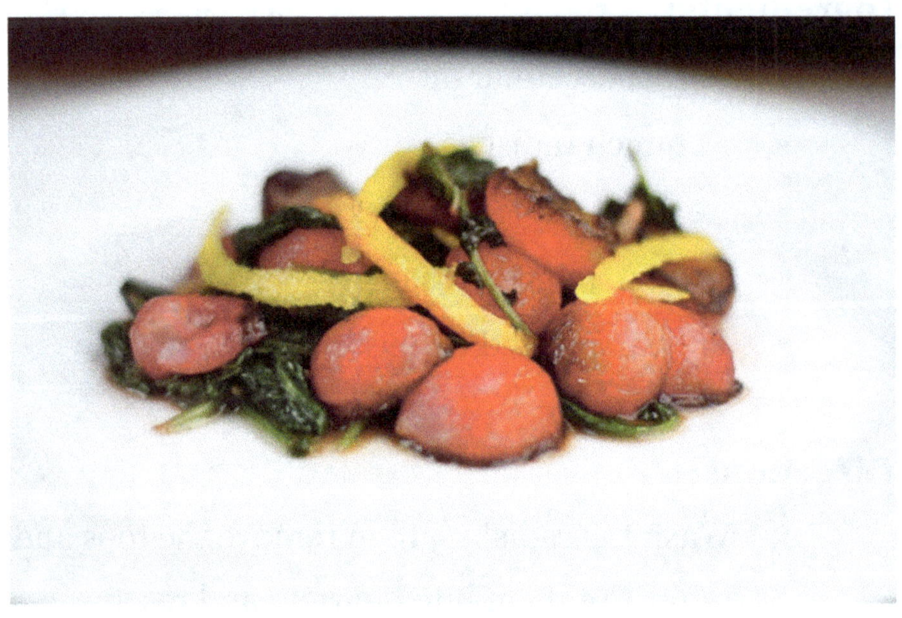

Rib Eyes With Broccoli

Servings: 4

Cooking Time: 15 Minutes

Ingredients:

- 4 ounces butter
- ¾ pound Ribeye steak, sliced
- 9 ounces broccoli, chopped
- 1 yellow onion, sliced
- 1 tablespoon coconut aminos
- 1 tablespoon pumpkin seeds
- Salt and pepper to taste

Directions:

1. Slice steak and the onions
2. Chop broccoli, including the stem parts
3. Take a frying pan and place it over medium heat, add butter and let it melt
4. Add meat and season accordingly with salt and pepper
5. Cook until both sides are browned

6. Transfer meat to a platter

7. Add broccoli and onion to the frying pan, add more butter if needed

8. Brown

9. Add coconut aminos and return the meat

10. Stir and season again

11. Serve with a dollop of butter with a sprinkle of pumpkin seeds

12. Enjoy!

Nutrition Info: Calories: 875 Fat: 75g Carbohydrates: 8g Protein: 40g

Salmon, Quinoa, And Avocado Salad

Servings: 4

Cooking Time: 20 Minutes

Ingredients:

- ½ cup quinoa
- 1 cup water
- 4 (4-ounce) salmon fillets
- 1-pound asparagus, trimmed
- 1 teaspoon extra-virgin olive oil, plus 2 tablespoons
- ½ teaspoon salt, divided
- ½ teaspoon freshly ground black pepper, divided
- ¼ teaspoon red pepper flakes
- 1 avocado, chopped
- ¼ cup chopped scallions, both white and green parts
- ¼ cup chopped fresh cilantro
- 1 tablespoon minced fresh oregano

- Juice of 1 lime

Directions:

1. In a small pot, combine the quinoa and water, and bring to a boil over medium-high heat. Cover, reduce the heat, and simmer for 15 minutes.

2. Preheat the oven to 425°F. Line a large baking sheet with parchment paper.

3. Arrange the salmon on one side of the prepared baking sheet. Toss the asparagus with 1 teaspoon of olive oil, and arrange on the other side of the baking sheet. Season the salmon and asparagus with ¼ teaspoon of salt, ¼ teaspoon of pepper, and the red pepper flakes. Roast for 12 minutes until browned and cooked through.

4. While the fish and asparagus are cooking, in a large mixing bowl, gently toss the cooked quinoa, avocado, scallions, cilantro, and oregano. Add the remaining 2 tablespoons of olive oil and the lime juice, and season with

the remaining ¼ teaspoon of salt and ¼ teaspoon of pepper.

5. Break the salmon into pieces, removing the skin and any bones, and chop the asparagus into bite-sized pieces. Fold into the quinoa and serve warm or at room temperature.

Nutrition Info: Calories: 397 Total Fat: 22g Protein: 29g Carbohydrates: 23g Sugars: 3g Fiber: 8g Sodium: 292mg

Orange Scallions And Brussels Sprouts

Servings: 4

Cooking Time: 25 Minutes

Ingredients:

- pound Brussels sprouts, trimmed and halved
- 1 cup scallions, chopped
- Zest of 1 lime, grated
- tablespoon olive oil
- ¼ cup orange juice
- tablespoons stevia
- A pinch of salt and black pepper

Directions:

1. Heat up a pan with the oil over medium heat, add the scallions and sauté for 5 minutes.
2. Add the sprouts and the other ingredients, toss, cook over medium heat for 20 minutes

more, divide the mix between plates and serve.

Nutrition Info: Calories 193 Fat 4 Fiber 1 Carbs 8 Protein 10

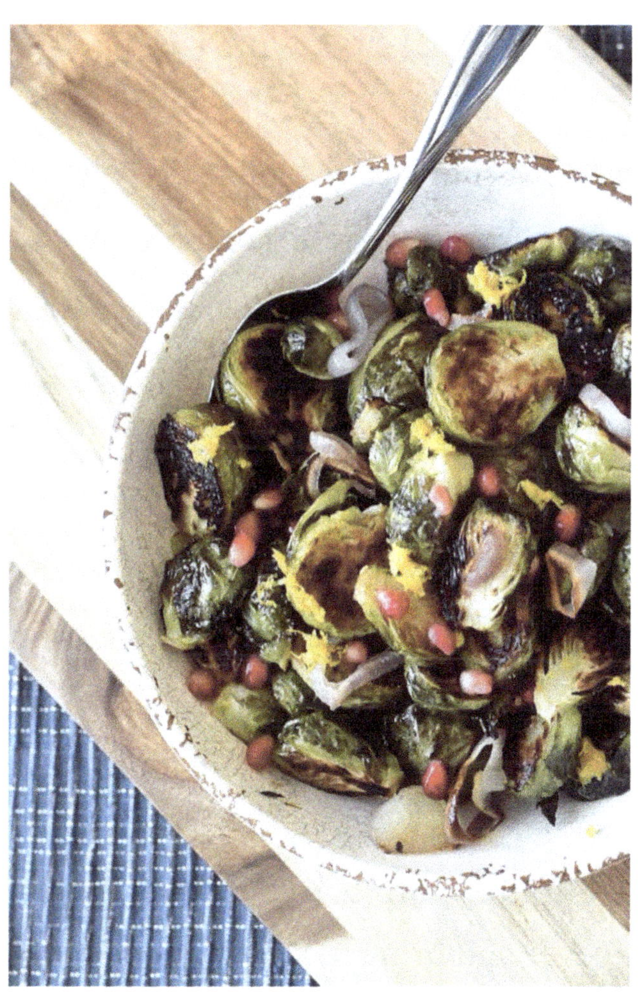

Carrot Ginger Soup

Servings: 4

Cooking Time: 20 Minutes

Ingredients:

- 1 tablespoon olive oil
- 1 medium yellow onion, chopped
- 3 cups fat-free chicken broth
- 1 pound carrots, peeled and chopped
- 1 tablespoon fresh grated ginger
- ¼ cup fat-free sour cream
- Salt and pepper

Directions:

1. Heat the oil in a large saucepan over medium heat.
2. Add the onions and sauté for 5 minutes until softened.
3. Stir in the broth, carrots, and ginger then cover and bring to a boil
4. Reduce heat and simmer for 20 minutes.

5. Stir in the sour cream then remove from heat.

6. Blend using an immersion blender until smooth and creamy.

7. Season with salt and pepper to taste then serve hot.

Nutrition Info: Calories 125, Total Fat 3.6g, Saturated Fat 0.5g, Total Carbs 17.2g, Net Carbs 13.6g, Protein 6.4g, Sugar 7.8g, Fiber 3.6g, Sodium 385mg

Shrimp And Black Bean Salad

Servings: 6

Cooking Time: None

Ingredients:

- ¼ cup apple cider vinegar
- 3 tablespoons olive oil
- 1 teaspoon ground cumin
- ½ teaspoon chipotle chili powder
- ¼ teaspoon salt
- 1 pound cooked shrimp, peeled and deveined
- 1 (15-ounce) can black beans, rinsed and drained
- 1 cup diced tomatoes
- 1 small green pepper, diced
- ¼ cup sliced green onions
- ¼ cup fresh chopped cilantro

Directions:

1. Whisk together the vinegar, olive oil, cumin, chili powder, and salt in a large bowl.
2. Chop the shrimp into bite-sized pieces then add to the bowl.
3. Toss in the beans, tomatoes, bell pepper, green onion, and cilantro until well combined.
4. Cover and chill until ready to serve.

Nutrition Info: Calories 405, Total Fat 9.5g, Saturated Fat 1.7g, Total Carbs 47.8g, Net Carbs 36.2, Protein 33.1, Sugar 2.8g, Fiber 11.6g, Sodium 291mg

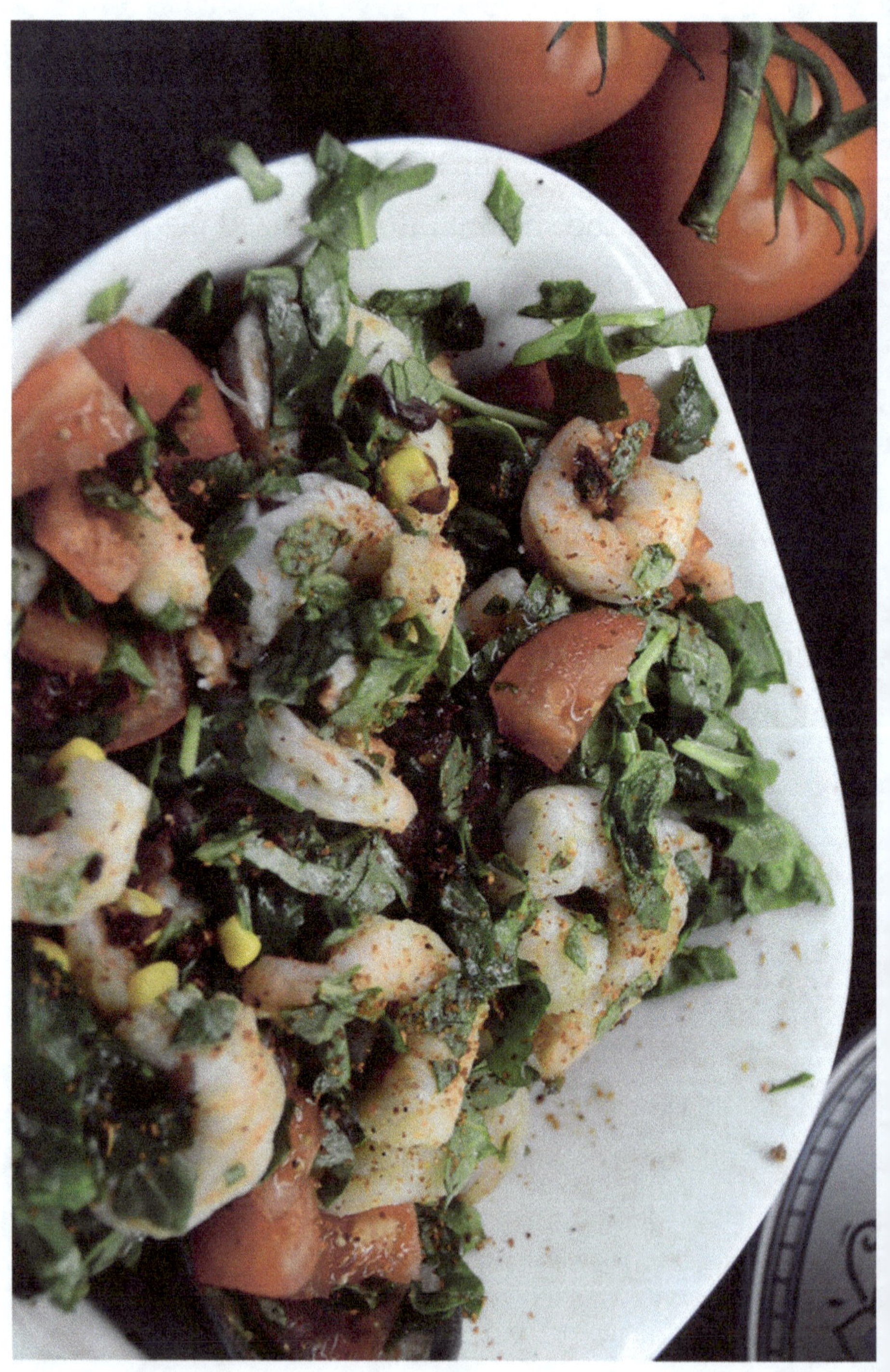

Spinach & Orange Salad

Servings: 6

Cooking Time: 0 Minutes

Ingredients:

- ¼ -1/3 Cup Vegan Dressing
- 3 Oranges, Medium, Peeled, Seeded & Sectioned
- ¾ lb. Spinach, Fresh & Torn
- 1 Red Onion, Medium, Sliced & Separated into Rings

Directions:

1. Toss everything together, and serve with dressing.
2. Interesting Facts: Spinach is one of the most superb green veggies out there. Each serving is packed with 3 grams of protein and is a highly encouraged component of the plant-based diet.

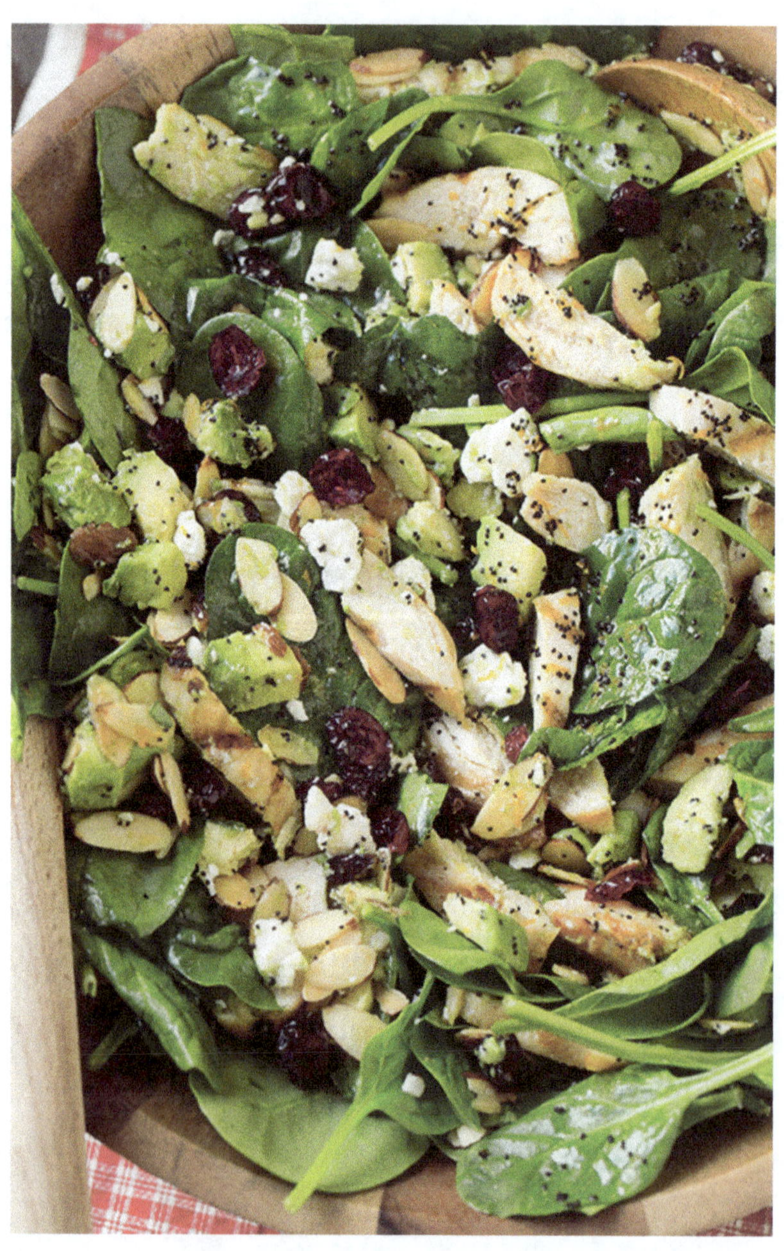

Bacon And Blue Cheese Salad

Servings: 2

Cooking Time: 5-7 Minutes

Ingredients:

- 2 and ½ ounces fresh spinach
- 1 red onion, sliced
- 3-4 tablespoons blue cheese, crumbled
- 2 ounces almond nibs
- 5 ounces bacon strips

Directions:

1. Fry bacon for 2-3 minutes each side, cut the bacon and keep it on the side
2. Take your salad plate and place spinach leaves on the bottom
3. Add sliced onion, cheese, bacon
4. Top with almond nibs
5. Use your desired Keto-Friendly salad dressing if needed
6. Toss and enjoy it!

Nutrition   Info: Calories: 420   Fat: 35g Carbohydrates: 2g Protein: 24g

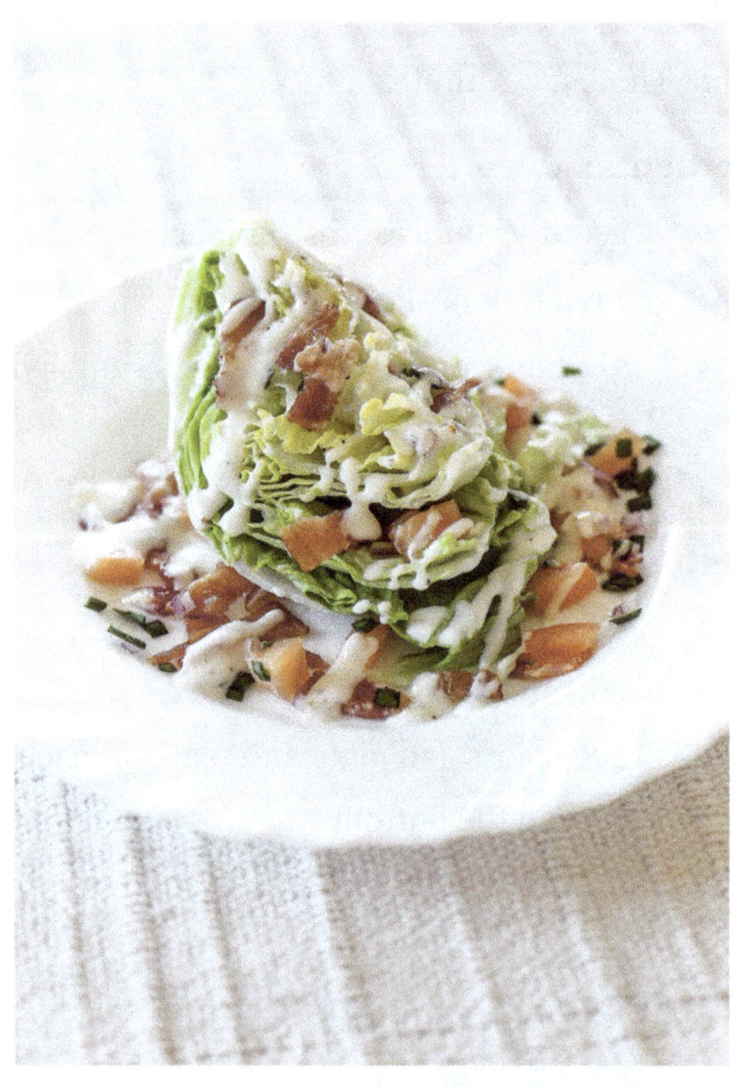

Baked Salmon Cakes

Servings: 4

Cooking Time: 20 Minutes

Ingredients:

- 15 ounces canned salmon, drained
- 1 large egg, whisked
- 2 teaspoons Dijon mustard
- 1 small yellow onion, minced
- 1 ½ cups whole-wheat breadcrumbs
- ¼ cup low-fat mayonnaise
- ¼ cup nonfat Greek yogurt, plain
- 1 tablespoon fresh chopped parsley
- 1 tablespoon fresh lemon juice
- 2 green onions, sliced thin

Directions:

1. Preheat the oven to 450°F and line a baking sheet with parchment.
2. Flake the salmon into a medium bowl then stir in the egg and mustard.

3. Mix in the onions and breadcrumbs by hand, blending well, then shape into 8 patties.

4. Grease a large skillet and heat it over medium heat.

5. Add the patties and fry for 2 minutes on each side until browned.

6. Transfer the patties to the baking sheet and bake for 15 minutes or until cooked through.

7. Meanwhile, whisk together the remaining ingredients.

8. Serve the baked salmon cakes with the creamy herb sauce.

Nutrition Info: Calories 240, Total Fat 12.2g, Saturated Fat 1.4g, Total Carbs 9.3g, Net Carbs 7.8g, Protein 25g, Sugar 1.8g, Fiber 1.5g, Sodium 241mg

Lighter Shrimp Scampi

Servings: 4

Cooking Time: 15 Minutes

Ingredients:

- 11/2 pounds large peeled and deveined shrimp
- ¼ teaspoon salt
- 1/8 teaspoon freshly ground black pepper
- 2 tablespoons olive oil
- 1 shallot, chopped
- 2 garlic cloves, minced
- ¼ cup cooking white wine
- Juice of 1/2 lemon (1 tablespoon)
- 1/2 teaspoon sriracha
- 2 tablespoons unsalted butter, at room temperature
- ¼ cup chopped fresh parsley
- 4 servings (6 cups) zucchini noodles with lemon vinaigrette

Directions:

1. Season the shrimp with the salt and pepper.

2. In a medium saucepan over medium heat, heat the oil. Add the shallot and garlic, and cook until the shallot softens and the garlic is fragrant, about 3 minutes. Add the shrimp, cover, and cook until opaque, 2 to 3 minutes on each side. Using a slotted spoon, transfer the shrimp to a large plate.

3. Add the wine, lemon juice, and sriracha to the saucepan, and stir to combine. Bring the mixture to a boil, then reduce the heat and simmer until the liquid is reduced by about half, 3 minutes. Add the butter and stir until melted, about 3 minutes. Return the shrimp to the saucepan and toss to coat. Add the parsley and stir to combine.

4. Into each of 4 containers, place 11/2 cups of zucchini noodles with lemon vinaigrette, and top with ¾ cup of scampi.

Nutrition Info: calories: 364; total fat: 21g; saturated fat: 6g; protein: 37g; total carbs: 10g; fiber: 2g; sugar: 6g; sodium: 557mg

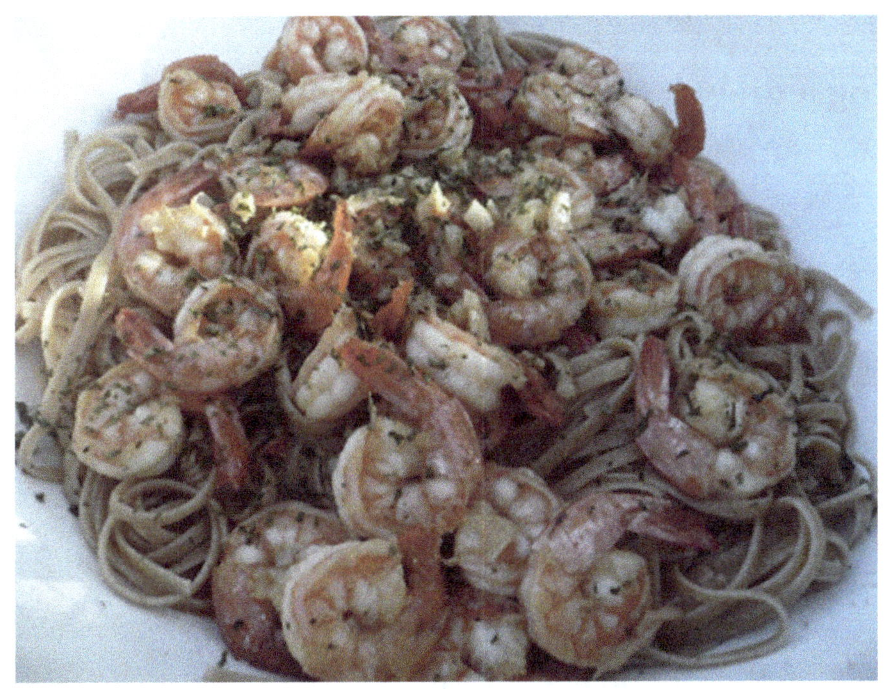

Onion And Bacon Pork Chops

Servings: 4

Cooking Time: 45 Minutes

Ingredients:

- 2 onions, peeled and chopped
- 6 bacon slices, chopped
- ½ cup chicken stock
- Salt and pepper to taste
- 4 pork chops

Directions:

1. Heat up a pan over medium heat and add bacon
2. Stir and cook until crispy
3. Transfer to bowl
4. Return pan to medium heat and add onions, season with salt and pepper
5. Stir and cook for 15 minutes
6. Transfer to the same bowl with bacon

7. Return the pan to heat (medium-high) and add pork chops

8. Season with salt and pepper and brown for 3 minutes

9. Flip and lower heat to medium

10. Cook for 7 minutes more

11. Add stock and stir cook for 2 minutes

12. Return the bacon and onions to the pan and stir cook for 1 minute

13. Serve and enjoy!

Nutrition Info: Calories: 325 Fat: 18g Carbohydrates: 6g Protein: 36g

Shrimp & Artichoke Skillet

Servings: 4

Cooking Time: 10 Minutes

Ingredients:

- 1 ½ cups shrimp, peel & devein
- 2 shallots, diced
- 1 tbsp. margarine
- What you'll need from store cupboard
- 2 12 oz. jars artichoke hearts, drain & rinse
- 2 cups white wine
- 2 cloves garlic, diced fine

Directions:

1. Melt margarine in a large skillet over med-high heat. Add shallot and garlic and cook until they start to brown, stirring frequently.
2. Add artichokes and cook 5 minutes. Reduce heat and add wine. Cook 3 minutes, stirring occasionally.

3. Add the shrimp and cook just until they turn pink. Serve.

Nutrition Info: Calories 487 Total Carbs 26g Net Carbs 17g Protein 64g Fat 5g Sugar 3g Fiber 9g

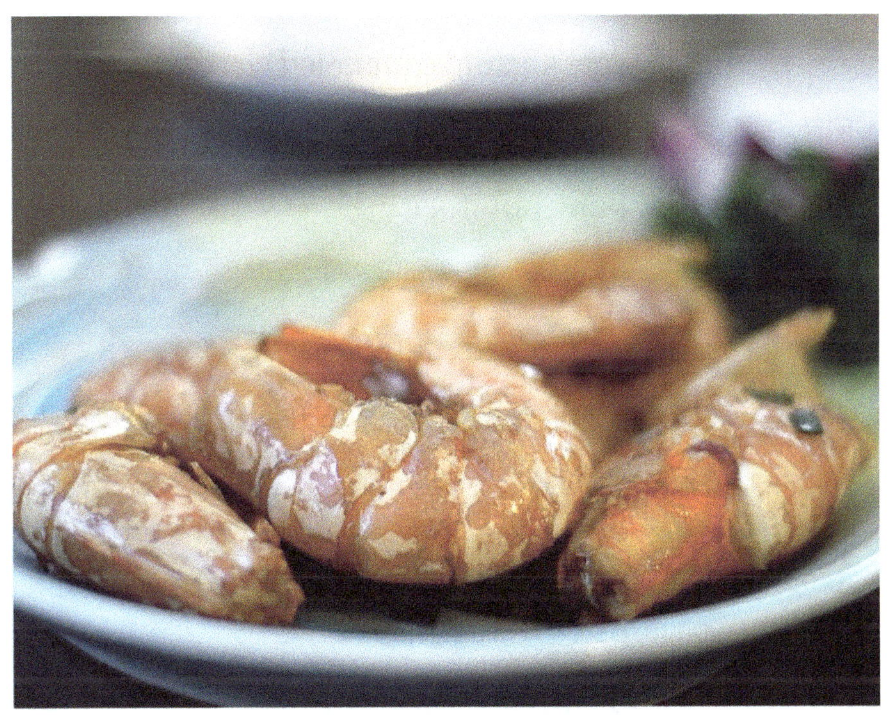

Shrimp Boil

Servings: 4

Cooking Time: 15 Minutes

Ingredients:

- 8 oz. raw shrimp, unpeeled
- 8 ooz. chicken sausage, small 1 inch pieces
- 8 oz. baby potatoes
- 1 sliced leek
- 2 corns, cut into half
- What you will need from the store cupboard:
- 3 tablespoons lemon juice
- 10 cups of water
- ¼ cup Old Bay seasoning
- Melted butter
- Lemon wedges

Directions:

1. Bring together the lemon juice, Old Bay, and water in your pot. Boil.
2. Include potatoes and cook for 5-7 minutes.
3. Add the sausage, shrimp, leek, and corn. Cook while stirring for another 5 minutes. The vegetables should be tender and the shrimp must be pink.
4. Now divide the vegetables, sausage, and shrimp with spoon and tongs among the serving bowls.
5. Drizzle the cooking liquid equally.
6. Serve with butter (optional).

Nutrition Info: Calories 202, Carbohydrates 22g, Fiber 2g, Sugar 0g, Cholesterol 109mg, Total Fat 5g, Protein 19g

Red Clam Sauce & Pasta

Servings: 4

Cooking Time: 3 Hours,

Ingredients:

- 1 onion, diced
- ¼ cup fresh parsley, diced
- What you'll need from store cupboard:
- 2 6 ½ oz. cans clams, chopped, undrained
- 14 ½ oz. tomatoes, diced, undrained
- 6 oz. tomato paste
- 2 cloves garlic, diced
- 1 bay leaf
- 1 tbsp. sunflower oil
- 1 tsp Splenda
- 1 tsp basil
- ½ tsp thyme
- ½ Homemade Pasta, cook & drain

Directions:

1.   Heat oil in a small skillet over med-high heat. Add onion and cook until tender, Add garlic and cook 1 minute more. Transfer to crock pot.

2.   Add remaining Ingredients, except pasta, cover and cook on low 3-4 hours.

3.   Discard bay leaf and serve over cooked pasta.

Nutrition Info: Calories 223 Total Carbs 32g Net Carbs 27g Protein 12g Fat 6g Sugar 15g Fiber 5g

Grilled Herbed Salmon With Raspberry Sauce & Cucumber Dill Dip

Servings: 4

Cooking Time: 30 Minutes

Ingredients:

- 3 salmon fillets
- 1 tablespoon olive oil
- Salt and pepper to taste
- 1 teaspoon fresh sage, chopped
- 1 tablespoon fresh parsley, chopped
- 2 tablespoons apple juice
- 1 cup raspberries
- 1 teaspoon Worcestershire sauce
- 1 cup cucumber, chopped
- 2 tablespoons light mayonnaise
- ½ teaspoon dried dill

Directions:

1. Coat the salmon fillets with oil.
2. Season with salt, pepper, sage and parsley.
3. Cover the salmon with foil.
4. Grill for 20 minutes or until fish is flaky.
5. While waiting, mix the apple juice, raspberries and Worcestershire sauce.
6. Pour the mixture into a saucepan over medium heat.
7. Bring to a boil and then simmer for 8 minutes.
8. In another bowl, mix the rest of the ingredients.
9. Serve salmon with raspberry sauce and cucumber dip.

Nutrition Info: Calories 256 Total Fat 15 g Saturated Fat 3 g Cholesterol 68 mg Sodium 176 mg Total Carbohydrate 6 g Dietary Fiber 1 g Total Sugars 5 g Protein 23 g Potassium 359 mg

Shrimp With Green Beans

Servings: 4

Cooking Time: 2 Minutes

Ingredients:

- ¾ pound fresh green beans, trimmed
- 1 pound medium frozen shrimp, peeled and deveined
- 2 tablespoons fresh lemon juice
- 2 tablespoons olive oil
- Salt and ground black pepper, as required

Directions:

1. Arrange a steamer trivet in the Instant Pot and pour cup of water.
2. Arrange the green beans on top of trivet in a single layer and top with shrimp.
3. Drizzle with oil and lemon juice.
4. Sprinkle with salt and black pepper.
5. Close the lid and place the pressure valve to "Seal" position.

6. Press "Steam" and just use the default time of 2 minutes.

7. Press "Cancel" and allow a "Natural" release.

8. Open the lid and serve.

Nutrition Info: Calories: 223, Fats: 1g, Carbs: 7.9g, Sugar: 1.4g, Proteins: 27.4g, Sodium: 322mg

Crab Curry

Servings: 2

Cooking Time: 20 Minutes

Ingredients:

- 0.5lb chopped crab
- 1 thinly sliced red onion
- 0.5 cup chopped tomato
- 3tbsp curry paste
- 1tbsp oil or ghee

Directions:

1. Set the Instant Pot to sauté and add the onion, oil, and curry paste.
2. When the onion is soft, add the remaining ingredients and seal.
3. Cook on Stew for 20 minutes.
4. Release the pressure naturally.

Nutrition Info: Calories 2; Carbs 11; Sugar 4; Fat 10; Protein 24; GL 9

Mussels In Tomato Sauce

Servings: 4

Cooking Time: 3 Minutes

Ingredients:

- 2 tomatoes, seeded and chopped finely
- 2 pounds mussels, scrubbed and de-bearded
- 1 cup low-sodium chicken broth
- 1 tablespoon fresh lemon juice
- 2 garlic cloves, minced

Directions:

1. In the pot of Instant Pot, place tomatoes, garlic, wine and bay leaf and stir to combine.
2. Arrange the mussels on top.
3. Close the lid and place the pressure valve to "Seal" position.
4. Press "Manual" and cook under "High Pressure" for about 3 minutes.

5. Press "Cancel" and carefully allow a "Quick" release.

6. Open the lid and serve hot.

Nutrition Info: Calories 213, Fats 25.2g, Carbs 11g, Sugar 1. Proteins 28.2g, Sodium 670mg